I0436191

EAT WELL
and
LOSE WEIGHT!

Written by: SHEILA BER-
Naturopathic Consultant.

INTRODUCTION:

I'm a Microbiological/Chemical Technologist, who is currently working as a Naturopathic Consultant.

I'm writing this book to provide advice and help, to treat overweight problems, by removing the root causes, rather than addressing the symptom only.

There are many internal and external factors, influencing the body and effecting how you feel, think, act, as well as how and what you eat.

Much of the advice provided in this book, is from my micro-biological/chemical background and experience, as well as own personal experience.

I dedicate the book to both my sons: Bernard and Philip. The book is dedicated also to all who seek help, and better their lives by examining first, at a <u>fundamental level,</u> all the contributing factors to their health problems, that consequently lead them to be overweight.

INDEX:

My best advice to you:

There are many solutions, and no one solution works on its own.
Our body chemistry is very individually complex, and one needs to consider all internal and external factors influencing our body. Therefore there is no one magic bullet that is safe to lose weight rapidly.

Multiple solutions, together will achieve synergistic, helpful and lasting effect when attempting to lose the extra weight.

2. The Dietary Guidelines for distribution of energy nutrients are as follows:

Fat: 30% of total calories
Protein: 25%
Carbohydrates: 45%

Carbs, short for carbohydrates, are a ready and easy supply of energy since they break down quickly. Most carbs will digest completely in about two hours. With that in mind, you should eat carbs that are <u>high in fiber</u> to slow the rush of sugar to the blood stream.

Proteins should be eaten in portions about the size of a deck of cards. Three to four of these portions will provide 60-80 grams (2.1 to 2.8 ounces) of the protein needed each day. If you're trying to build muscle, it's a good idea to add a few more grams of protein each day to promote muscle growth.

Saturated fats are not as heart healthy as mono-unsaturated or polyunsaturated fats, but they are important and as much as 10% of your fat intake can come from saturated fats. They are mostly animal fats, including fat from dairy products.

Minimize their consumption, and if you consume more than recommended, you can cancel out saturated fats, by following the steps described below, in clause #7.

1. What is pH?

pH is an acronym for the "potential of Hydrogen", or the acid to alkaline ratio existing in all matter, and our 7.365 body pH measurement is the benchmark for measuring our health.

Our pH normal range value can be likened to our body's temperature; we each have a normal range value of 98.6 degrees. When our body temperature increases or decreases we typically experience symptoms, and more importantly, we also know there is an underlying reason when our temperature is not normal.

pH scale measures acid to alkaline: 0 to 14.

Our body pH should be 7.365, which is considered neutral.

7.365 being neutral, if your pH is 6.365 - you are 10x more acidic than normal range.

7.365 being neutral, if your pH is 5.365 - you are 100x more acidic than normal range.

*You can see how the pH factor compounds itself. This is why people will feel as though their health has spiraled, and thus are required to take action to normalize their pH balance. Please refer to clause #9.

3. To achieve maximum results, in attempting to lose weight, you <u>must first tackle all the health aspects</u> as following:

-<u>Physically</u>: Exercise- without excessive exertion, body restoration such as: Yoga, massage, spa, etc.

- <u>Mentally</u>: Relaxation, mind restoration including Yoga, other effective ways of dealing with stress, and/or with any mental conditions, if present.

- <u>Spiritually</u>: Yoga, meditation, prayer, herbal treatments.

- <u>Chemically</u>: Supplements, vitamins, alkalizing agents (ie. Sodium Bicarbonate, also called Baking Soda) - used also for neutralizing body acidic pH, to maintain good health).

- <u>Microbially</u>: Probiotics, digestive enzymes, and the important daily elimination of microbial & chemical toxins.

- *Electrolytrically:* *Drinking daily: 6-8 glasses water. Also supplementing daily with Minerals to balance body electrolytes, as follows: Sodium, Potassium, Magnesium, and Calcium. These minerals are extremely important for: efficient metabolism and electrical conductivity, impacting every cell in your body, including the nervous system, all muscles, glands and organs. The BRAIN and the HEART are particularly affected, due to their higher electrical activity.*

*Optimal electrical conductivity, provides the body with better circulation, more energy, higher level of Oxygen, strong immune system, and improved bodily functions.

4. Have a underline blood test annually, or more often if required. Check with your family Doctor the important body levels as following:

  - *THYROID*
  - *HEMOGLOBIN*
  - *IRON*
  - *CORTISOL*
  - *CHOLESTEROL*
  - *HORMONES*
  - *ESR*

The reason all the above items have to be checked, is because the slightest imbalance in any one, will actually impede you from achieving your goal to lose weight, whether at a slow or at a faster rate.

If your <u>Thyroid</u> level is low, treat it!
You can also treat it naturally, by taking daily, Lugol Iodine:8 drops in some filtered water - 2x a day, for 2 months, on an empty stomach, and can continue treatment for an indefinite period: 8 drops - once a day.

If your <u>Hemoglobin</u> and <u>Iron</u> levels are low: 1) take daily 1-2 Iron capsules, from a <u>vegetable source</u> (a mild form that does not cause constipation). Take it with vitamin C - 500 mg, for optimum absorption. 2) Take B-12: 1000-5000 mcg. <u>Methyl</u>cobalamine version, which helps assimilate much better.

If your <u>Cortisol</u> level is high, its indicatory of your high stress level, and you can treat it naturally, by taking the following supplements:

1) B-Complex 1-2 tablets daily,

2) L-Theanine (Amino acid) 500 mg. 1-2x a day. It helps to reduce anxiety. It is commonly found in Green tea.

3) Holy Basil 500 mg. also helps with anxiety.

4) Passion flower <u>extract</u> or <u>capsules</u>: 1-3x daily for about 30 days, and stop. Take this herb only during period of extreme stress and anxiety.

5. <u>Ladies</u>: check your <u>hormone</u> levels of: Estrogen, Progesterone, DHEA and Testosterone.

<u>Gentlemen</u>: check your <u>hormone</u> levels of: Testosterone, Estrogen and DHEA.

If your Estrogen level is high, you are <u>Estrogen dominant</u>. You then <u>need to balance your hormones</u>, by getting a bioidentical Progesterone cream 3%-6%, and applying it daily on your skin.

It is applied once daily, alternating skin areas: abdomen, front neck, inside mid arms, inside and back of thighs.

Bioidentical form of Progesterone assimilates more efficiently, delivers fast results, and is safer!

It is produced from a natural source.

Progesterone will make you feel better, more calm, and will also help balance your thyroid, and all other systems in your body. Even your sleep will be better.

For more information you can go to:

http://www.hystersisters.com/vb2/article_97232.htm

and

http://www.livestrong.com/article/228083-benefits-of-bioidentical-hormones/

*Estrogen dominance can pose a high risk for developing cancer, if not treated in due course. Some of the many side effects are, <u>overeating</u>, sugar cravings, and higher aggression, in both women and men.

If your <u>ESR</u> level is high, it is indicatory of <u>high inflammation</u> level in the body. Treat it- if it is high!

You can take a tablet of coated Baby Aspirin 81 mg. to reduce the inflammation effectively, daily or every other day.

Also during weight loss, ESR level fluctuates, so it is recommended to have a blood test every 3-6 months, to address any abnormality.

6) a) Reduce consumption of saturated fats to a minimum. That being said, our body definitely needs a certain amount, to function optimally. For diets that are too rich in saturated fats, see my suggestions in clause #7, to cancel them out!

b) Exercise 15-30 minutes daily. NEVER overexert yourself! It is unhealthy and stressful. <u>Stress will elevate your Cortisol level</u>, which will actually cause you to gain weight, and thus it is counterproductive.

  c) *Periodically, alternate the type of exercises that you do.*
*The muscles that you work out eventually get desensitized
and will have lower resistance.*

**Remember: you burn calories faster, when your muscles
have higher resistance, during the exercise:*

*HIGHER MUSCLE RESISTANCE= HIGHER NO. OF
CALORIES BURNED,*
and
*LOWER MUSCLE RESISTANCE= LOWER NO. OF
CALORIES BURNED.*

and

*HIGHER INTENSITY EXERCISE is not always equal to
HIGHER MUSCLE RESISTANCE, and thus will not
always burn you more calories.*

Working out longer, and more intensely, with muscles that no longer have high resistance, again will have you burn less calories than when you burned previously, when your muscles had higher resistance.

For this reason, it is recommended that you alternate any set of exercises that you do, every few days. Also change the duration time, and intensity level, so that your body does not get desensitized completely to any particular set of exercises.

7. TO CANCEL OUT SATURATED FATS (including CARBS, SUGARS:

Daily take the following:

a) 1-2 spoons EXTRA VIRGIN COCONUT OIL (you can purchase it at Healthy Planet Health store), and you can also take 1 tablespoon EXTRA VIRGIN OLIVE OIL (high quality, such as "Evoo").

Yes! These oils will balance your HDL/LDL levels, due to the special chemical composition that they both acquire.

***HDL** *definition: High Density Lipid (good cholesterol)*

***LDL** *" : Low Density Lipid (saturated fats – bad cholesterol).*

b) 2-3 capsules 1000 mg. LECITHIN. It also comes in granules, so take 2x daily, 2 tablespoons daily, in soups, teas, or juices. Lecithin is an emulsifier! It therefore helps emulsify fats. It is also beneficial for the brain, heart, and liver. It helps with memory. It is also great to induce sleep.

c) 1 spoon FLAX OIL.

d) 2-4 spoons COD LIVER OIL (also high in Omega).

e) 2 spoons APPLE CIDER VINEGAR in 1 cup warm water, especially after a heavy or fatty meal.

f) Take PROBIOTICS! They aid in digestion, reduce inflammation, enhance metabolism. 1-2 capsules once or twice daily, 1/2 hr. before meals, with a glass of warm water. Probiotics also help with treating yeast infections.

g) Take ENZYMES 2-3x daily, with meals, for complete digestion, optimum metabolism, treating yeast infection, and allergies. Enzymes digest putrid matter in your digestive system, and also digest microbes, yeast, and even cancer cells.

How Do You Know if You Are Lacking Enzymes?

Heartburn, gas, constipation, bloating, allergies, ulcers, lack of energy and reduced functioning of the immune system, may occur when there are not enough enzymes.

*8. **PLEASE NOTE:* **Yeasty foods and drinks can be addictive!** *When you eat or drink yeasty foods, drinks, such as: PIZZA, PASTRY, WINE, BEER,* *consume in moderation, and immediately take <u>**Probiotics**</u>, to get rid of the excessive yeast in your body. <u>Probiotics digest yeast, consequently they help reduce your cravings to foods that contain yeast!!!</u>*

9. <u>BAKING SODA</u> (Arm & Hammer) – <u>to neutralize your body acidic pH</u>, to maintain good health, higher energy level, and efficient oxygenation - Take 1/2 tsp Baking Soda, in 1 glass water, along with POTASSIUM - one capsule <u>99 mg</u>. (to balance the electrolytes in your body, by maintaining Sodium/Potassium ratio balanced).

<u>Note</u>: You must take the drink with the Potassium, in order <u>to also maintain a normal blood pressure</u>.

Baking Soda (2NaHCO3): Aids digestion, provides energy, slows/reduces microbial activity, alkalizes your body due to the 3 Oxygen atoms in the soda, thus better in neutralizing your body acidic pH.

 An acidic diet is comprised of high percentage of sugars, carbohydrates, proteins and fats. It is probably low or lacking in vegetables and fruits.

Body acidic pH is due to an acidic diet, and particularly also, due to high level of stress.

*Body acidic pH will render you tired, sluggish, low or deprived in oxygen, resulting in higher microbial activity, increase in inflammation level, and at a greater risk of developing cancer. This is because CANCER thrives and grows only in an acidic environment!!!

*Keep your body pH always slightly alkaline at: 7.0 - 7.5!!!

Follow instructions to alkalize, as in clause #9 above.

10. BODY DAILY ELIMINATION of Microbial and Chemical TOXINS:
Daily elimination of toxins is crucial for good health.

If you are occasionally encountering a problem eliminating, you can try one, or more of the following suggestions:

a) Eat a healthy amount of vegetables, whole grains and beans to get a variety of <u>fibers, vitamins and minerals</u>.

b) Drink plenty of filtered water: 6-8 glasses of water daily.

c) Take Probiotics, 1-2 capsules on empty stomach, with 1 cup of <u>warm</u> water, 20 minutes before breakfast, and also before bed.

d) Eat several prunes, to help with stool softening, and quicker bowel motility.

e) Add Lecithin granules: 1 spoon, in your coffee, tea, or food. It works especially, when you add it to a warm/hot liquid. Alternately, you can take 1 capsule 2x daily with warm water.

f) Add 1-2 tablespoons of ground <u>Flax seeds</u> into 1/2 cup of boiled water, stir, leave for a minute, add 1/2 cup lukewarm water, and drink, preferably on empty stomach.

It helps with a smoother movement. It is rich in Omega oil.

g) Drink special HERBAL LAXATIVE TEA (excellent brand is: Triple Leaf). It will give you gentle effective relief, especially if you drink it hot, on empty stomach, 1/2 hour before a meal.

NOTE: *If none of the above was of any help, then you may have parasites, that cause stubborn constipation, and it would therefore be best that you consult with a Naturopathic Doctor, who can give you a simple test, to determine if you do have them.

If you do, you'll be given a simple herbal treatment, to take for about 20 days. The treatment is safe, easy, simple, and effective.

*I can recommend anyone an excellent Naturopathic Doctor: Dr. Diana Enzo, at: 905-477-0200, Address: 3160 Steeles Ave. E. (just W. of Victoria Park Ave.), in Toronto, Ontario, Canada. He has many years of experience behind him, and is very reliant.

If you have parasites and you don't seek treatment to eliminate them, you may experience a continuing constipation problem, along with many other undesirable health problems. To find out if you have parasites, ask yourself the following questions:

DO I EXPERIENCE THE FOLLOWING:

Constipation: Some worms, because of their shape and large size, can physically obstruct certain organs. Heavy worm infections can block the common bile duct and the intestinal tract, making elimination infrequent and difficult.

Diarrhoea: Certain parasites, primarily protozoa, produce a prostaglandin (hormone like substance) found in various human tissues) which creates a sodium and chloride loss that leads to frequent watery stools.

The diarrhoea process in parasite infection is, therefore, a function of the parasite, not the body's attempt to rid itself of an infectious organism.

Gas and Bloating: Some parasites live in the upper small intestine where the inflammation they produce causes both gas and bloating. The situation can be magnified when hard-to-digest foods such as beans and raw fruits and vegetables are eaten. Persistent abdominal distention is a frequent sign of hidden invaders.

These gastrointestinal symptoms can persist intermittently for many months or years if the parasites are not eliminated from the body.

Irritable bowel syndrome: Parasites can irritate inflame, coal, the intestinal cell wall, leading to a variety of gastrointestinal symptoms and malabsorption of vital nutrients, particularly fatty substances. This malabsorption leads to bulky stools and steatorrhea (excess fat in feces)

Joint and muscle aches and pains: *Parasites are known to migrate to encyst (become enclosed in a sac) in joint fluids, and worms can encyst in muscles. Once that happens, pain becomes evident and is often assumed to be caused by arthritis Joint, and muscle pains and inflammation are also the result of tissue damage caused by some parasites of the body's ongoing immune response to then- presence.*

Anaemia: *Some varieties of intestinal worms attach themselves to the mucosal lining of the intestines and then leach nutrients from the human host.*

If they are present in large enough numbers, they can create enough blood loss to cause a type of iron deficiency or pernicious Anaemia.

Allergy: *Parasites can irritate and sometimes perforate the intestinal lining, increasing bowel permeability to large undigested molecules. This can activate the body's immune response to produce increased levels of Eosinophils, one type of the body's fighter cells.*

The Eosinophils can inflame body tissue, resulting in an allergic reaction. <u>Like allergy, parasites also trigger an increase in the production of immunoglobulin E (IgE).</u>

<u>Skin conditions</u>: Intestinal worms can cause hives, rashes, weeping eczema, and other allergic-type skin reactions. Cutaneous ulcers, swellings and sores, popular lesions, and itchy dermatitis can result from protozoan invasion.

<u>Granuloma</u>: Granulomas are tumour-like masses that encase destroyed large or parasitic eggs. They develop most often in the colon or rectal walls but can also be found in the lungs, liver, peritoneum, and uterus.

<u>Nervousness</u>: Parasitic metabolic wastes and toxic substances can serve as irritants to the central nervous system. Restlessness and anxiety are often the result of the systemic parasite infestation. (After completing a herbal cleanse, many people swear that their persistently grouchy mates or relatives have become a lot more pleasant and patient. "The most famous tapeworm of recent years belonged to the late opera singer Maria Callas.

She had a serious weight and skin problem. When the tapeworm was detected and removed, ha" weight dropped, her skin improved and her temperament mellowed," says Dr. Louise Gittleman, who was treating Ms. Callas.

Sleep disturbances: Multiple awakening during the night particularly between 2 and 3 AM, are possibly caused by the body's attempts to eliminate toxic wastes via the liver. According to Chinese medicine, these hours are governed by the liver. Sleep disturbances are also caused by nocturnal exits of certain parasites through the anus, creating the intense discomfort and itching.

Teeth grinding: Bruxism - abnormal grinding, clenching, and gnashing of the teeth - has been observed in cases of parasitic infection. These symptoms are most noticeable among children. Bruxism may be a nervous response to the internal foreign irritant.

Chronic fatigue: Chronic fatigue symptoms include tiredness, flu-like complaints, apathy, depression, impaired concentration, and faulty memory.

Parasites cause these physical, mental, and emotional symptoms through malnutrition resulting from malabsorption of proteins, carbohydrates, fats, and especially vitamins A and B-12.

Immune Dysfunction: Parasites depress immune system functioning by decreasing the secretion of immunoglobulin A (I&A).

Their presence continuously stimulates the system response and over time can exhaust this vital defense system, leaving the body open to bacterial and viral infections.

The following conditions might also be tell-tale signs of an invasion: weight gain, excessive hunger, weight loss, bad taste in the mouth and bad breath, asthma, diabetes, epilepsy, acne, migraines, and the biggest killers: heart disease and cancer.

*By examining all the above information closely, and by following the instructions, you will treat the root causes of your weight problems, and not just the symptoms.

Additionally, you will enjoy much better health.

I WISH YOU GOOD LUCK and GOOD HEALTH!

SHEILA BER, 2012.

DISCLAIMER.

Copyright © 2012 Sheila Ber. All rights reserved.

BIOGRAPHY 2012.

Professionally:

I'm a **Microbiological/Chemical Technologist**, currently working as a **Naturopathic consultant**.
I worked in Microbiology and Chemistry, for about 12 years, in the Pharmaceutical, cosmetics, and toiletry industries.

I started out as a microbiological/Chemical Analyst. I Performed: chemical and microbiological analysis of raw materials, finished products, variety of packaging materials and their compatibility with different range of finished products.
Chemical analysis tests were carried out with up to date technologically advanced instruments, such as Spectrophotometers, and other apparatus.

Microbiological tests including incubation of samples, and microscopical studies of a variety of bacteria, yeast, and fungus.

I was involved also in Research & Development, and in formulations of large variety of products.

I've advanced several years later, to a higher position with the title of Quality Control Manager.

My work included:

1) Quality Control of raw materials, finished products, and packaging.

2) I was responsible for managing and supporting the laboratory personnel.

3) Additionally, I have carried out inspections on the production floor facilities, the equipment, including ventilation system, and other systems. Monthly reporting on the findings, my recommendations, and implementation of required corrective actions.

4) Communication with Health Canada, particularly to obtain their regulatory approvals for new patents of new products. Provision of documentation, and MSDS information of the raw material involved, in all the formulations.

I have tremendously enjoyed all the above duties.

It's very technically involved work, very interesting, and challenging.

Personally:

Generally, I'm rather unconventional, though as getting older, I become slightly more conventional. I like things straight, simple, and uncomplicated.

I like helping people. I try to view things, situations, from different perspectives.

I refrain from judging others, but need to know all the facts and reasons for their particular behaviour, thoughts and actions, before forming any opinion.

Life has its highs and lows, but I always try to stay afloat. Trying is the key word!

I often check my expectations, and may lower them occasionally, to keep things in perspective.

At the age of 20, I've completed 2 years of service, in the Army, filling the position of Sergeant. It was definitely, a significant lifetime experience!

I have two grown up sons. I love them very dearly.

I enjoy being a caring mother, not perfect, and with always room for improve.

EDUCATION:

I've graduated with **Honours in Science,** and with **Distinction in Physics.**

Seneca College
Microbiological/Chemical Technology.

Technical school
Architecture/Mechanical Drafting.

School of Accounting
General Accounting.

OCCUPATION:

I'm currently working as a Naturopathic Consultant.

EMPLOYMENT HISTORY:

DRUG TRADING COMPANY - Toronto
Microbiological/Chemical Technologist.

FABERGE - Toronto
Quality Control - Laboratory Manager.

REVLON - Toronto
Quality Control - Laboratory Manager.

Accenture Business for Utilities - Toronto
Accounting/Administration.

Lived in:

1) Toronto, Canada,
2) Argentina.

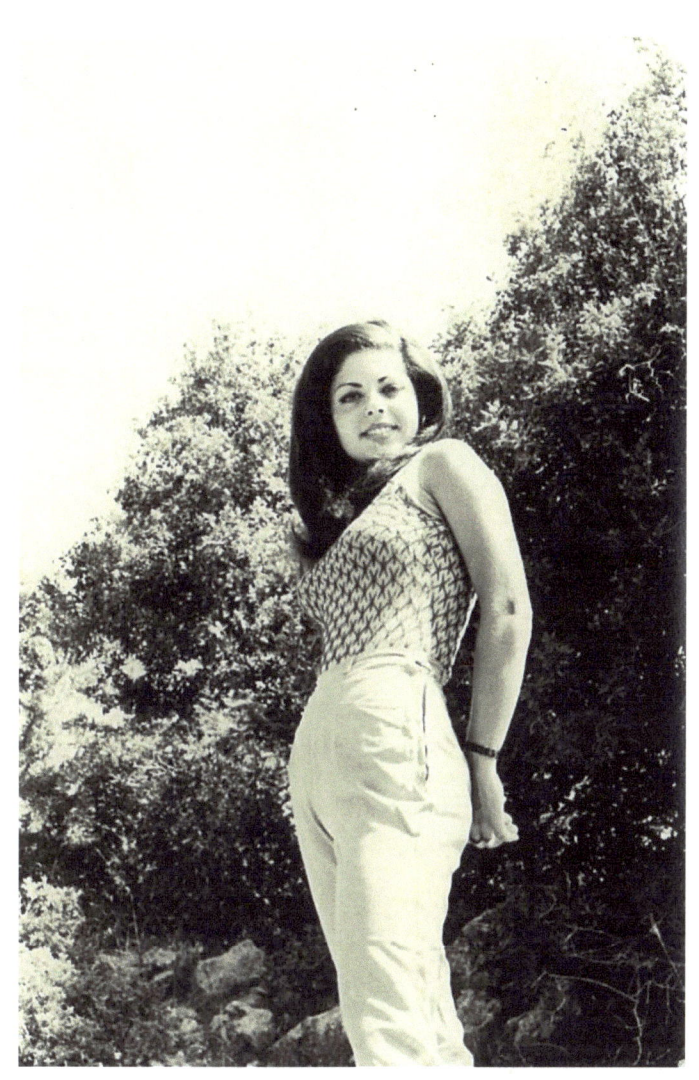

SHEILA BER, 2012.
(SHULLA)

Disclaimer.

Copyright © 2012 Sheila Ber. All rights reserved.

ALKALIZE and SURVIVE!

"Alkalize and Survive" book is also written by Sheila Ber,
at: *www.Amazon.com*
www.Createspace.com
www.Cobobooks.com
www.Indigo.Chapters.ca

www.ingramcontent.com/pod-product-compliance
Lightning Source LLC
Chambersburg PA
CBHW041530280526
45792CB00004B/1442